Coconut Oil

Rev Up Your System— Change Your Oil!

Barbara Wexler, M.P.H.

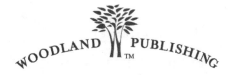

WOODLAND PUBLISHING ™

For permissions, ordering information, or bulk quantity discounts, please contact: Woodland Publishing, 448 East 800 North, Orem, Utah 84097
Visit our Web site: www.woodlandpublishing.com
Toll-free number: (800) 777-2665

Cataloging-in-Publication data available from the Library of Congress.

ISBN-13: 978-1-58054-464-1
ISBN-10: 1-58054-464-9

Printed in the United States of America

06   07   08   09   10   1   2   3   4   5   6   7   8   9   10

Contents

Rev Up Your System—Change Your Oil!

In the 1973 movie *Sleeper*, Woody Allen plays Miles Monroe, a mild-mannered guy who wakes up, befuddled, after accidentally being put to sleep by his doctors for two hundred years. Early in the movie, Miles tries to catch up with all the changes he missed, including the complete transformation of the social and political environment he once knew. And the biggest laugh comes when he discovers that the miracle health food of the future is—fat!

The idea that fat could be healthy seemed absurd back in 1973 and for most people, it still does today. We've been at war with fat for decades. We've struggled through a minefield of saturated fats, trans fats, oily foods, anything having to do with that awful, slimy, slippery stuff most of us try to lose—not consume.

But the tide is turning as scientists, doctors, and nutritionists have taken a deeper, more sophisticated look at the role of lipids—the scientific term that includes all fats and oils—in creating and maintaining health. It's now becoming widely accepted that certain oils like coconut oil and a variety of fish and seed oils provide substantial, sometimes astonishing, health benefits.

Did you know that:

- Every cell in your body is surrounded with a coating of oil—and that maintaining the proper composition of this oily membrane is one of the most important aspects of cellular health?
- Most of the energy that powers the body is made by burning lipids, called free fatty acids (FFAs), that are derived from fats and oil—and not sugar?
- Many metabolic disorders that seem to be about controlling blood sugar levels, like diabetes and hypoglycemia, may often be caused in large part by improper handling of fats?
- For most people, one of the best ways to lose weight is to improve how the body processes oils and fats—by actually eating more of the right kinds?
- The ratio of certain oils—called essential fatty acids (EFAs)—has a huge impact on either creating or reducing inflammatory disorders including arthritis, heart disease, and nervous system complaints?
- Lipids play an intimate role in the production of hormones that govern countless metabolic and biological processes from the perception of hunger to our responses to stress and the timing of our reproductive cycles?
- Some oils, like coconut oil, in addition to their nutritive properties, also have immune system benefits including powerful antiviral activity?
- Fats are essential to life? Properly selecting and balancing the fats and oils we consume is a key to unlocking the greatest gift of all—optimal health!

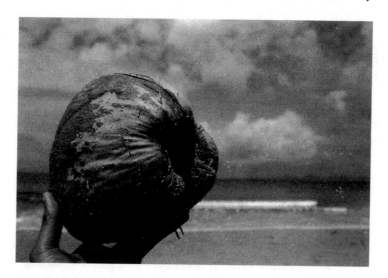

Healing From the Tree of Life

The pungent sweet scent of coconut oil conjures up visions of tall swaying palms in a lush tropical paradise. For many island communities and tropical regions around the world, coconut is a diet staple and the coconut palm, *Cocos nucifera*, is the staff of life, providing food and drink as well as cooking oil, body oil, and industrial oil. Almost one-third of the world's population—throughout South and Central America, Africa, India, Micronesia, Melanesia, Polynesia, and much of Asia—relies on the coconut palm as a source of food and sustenance.

The coconut palm is often referred to as a "three-generation tree," supporting the farmer, his children and grandchildren. It's also been called the "tree of life," or *kalpa vriksha*, in Sanskrit, which literally translated means "the tree which provides all the necessities of life." The traditional medicine practices among Asian and Pacific Islanders value the tree's oil as more than simply a powerful source of nutrition; they consider it a potent medicine, capable of healing a wide range of ailments.

About three-quarters of the world's coconut supply comes from India, where coconuts have been cultivated for more than three thousand years. Coconut is considered a divine plant in Vedic tradition and assumes a place of honor in sacred ceremonies. Ayurvedic (knowledge of life) medicine has a long history of using coconut oil as medicine. Ayurveda and traditional medicine used coconut oil to treat illnesses ranging from bronchitis, fever, and flu to thyroid disorders, tumors, and sexually transmitted diseases.

Today, coconut oil is used to ease digestive disorders in children and adults, to help people with skin problems such as psoriasis, and to speed the healing of cuts and burns. There is evidence that coconut oil may help to prevent osteoporosis—the decrease in bone mass and bone mineral density that increases the risk of fractures—by boosting absorption of minerals such as calcium and magnesium. In fact, because coconut oil improves absorption of many nutrients, enabling the body to readily use fat-soluble vitamins—A, D, E, K, beta-carotene, and some B vitamins—it has been used to successfully treat people suffering from malnutrition and is a key component of infant formula.

There also are promising reports of studies using coconut oil to help prevent liver and kidney diseases and Crohn's disease, a type of inflammatory bowel condition that causes sufferers to experience chronic abdominal pain. Other research describes the use of coconut oil's antimicrobial properties to help resolve infections—not only bacterial infections, but also yeast, fungal, and viral infections. Coconut oil contains lauric acid, which imparts its antimicrobial action. The very same antimicrobial properties likely account for coconut oil's ability to help improve dental health by preventing dental cavities.

Since coconut oil possesses antiviral properties, researchers are also looking at how it might be used to treat diseases such as infection with the herpes virus and HIV (human immunodeficiency virus)—the virus that causes AIDS, acquired immunodeficiency syndrome. At least one small pilot study reported promising results—that coconut oil has an antiviral effect that can beneficially reduce the viral load of HIV patients.

Other investigators have observed that coconut oil appears to offer some protection from cancer-causing chemicals known as muta-carcinogens such as benzypyrine, azaserine, and nitrosamines. Animal studies found strong evidence of coconut oil's protective effect compared to soybean oil. It not only offered protection when the animals consumed it as part of their diet for several days before they were exposed to the cancer-causing chemicals but also protected them when the cancer-causing chemical and coconut oil were consumed together.

A Broad Spectrum of Benefits

The compounds naturally found in coconut oil have been reported to possess a wide range of health benefits that enhance:

- Cardiovascular health—by lowering total cholesterol levels and improving the ratio of "good" HDL to "bad" LDL cholesterol
- Immune system health—by providing a broad range of antiviral, antibacterial, antifungal, and antiparasitic actions
- Metabolic health—by increasing the metabolic rate, supporting the burning of stored fat, and increasing the production of natural enzymes
- Physical and cosmetic skin health—by nourishing the skin, inhibiting infections, and offering some protection from damage by ultraviolet radiation
- Digestive health—by providing a quality source of cellular energy and improving the absorption and utilization of other important nutrients

In a bit more detail, here are some of the purported benefits of the various compounds found in coconut oil. Some of these reported benefits may come from using coconut oil for cooking and as a nutritional supplement. Other benefits may require the concentration of certain compounds derived from coconut oil, such as monolaurin, which has been reported to be a potent antiviral agent. This information is adapted from publications of the Coconut Research Center, Boulder, Colorado.

Coconut oil and its naturally associated compounds may:

- Offer a measure of antiviral activity helping to protect against influenza, herpes, measles, hepatitis C, SARS (severe acute respiratory syndrome), HIV, and other viruses
- Provide antibacterial activity helping to protect against various microbes implicated in conditions including ulcers, throat infections, urinary tract infections, gum disease and cavities, pneumonia, and gonorrhea
- Have antimycotic activity helping to protect against *Candida albicans* and other molds and yeasts associated with ringworm, athlete's foot, thrush, diaper rash, and other mycotic conditions
- Provide antiparasitic activity helping the body to kill or expel tapeworms, lice, giardia, and other parasites
- Deliver a rapidly available source of natural energy
- Enhance energy and endurance, which is especially important for physical and athletic performance
- Improve digestion and absorption of nutrients including vitamins, minerals, and amino acids
- Help reduce excess cholesterol and improve the ratio of high-density lipoproteins to low-density lipoproteins (HDL/LDL ratio). Research has shown that boosting this ratio may help reduce the risk of heart disease
- Protect arteries from the types of inflammatory damage associated with atherosclerosis and thereby help protect against heart disease
- Improve insulin mobilization and availability of glucose in the blood.

- Help support the body's natural production of enzymes
- Provide nutritional support for the symptoms and health risks of diabetes
- Have a positive impact on the absorption of calcium and magnesium, supporting the development of strong bones and teeth and reducing the risk of osteoporosis
- Relieve symptoms associated with gallbladder disease
- Help relieve symptoms associated with gastrointestinal disorders including Crohn's disease, ulcerative colitis, and stomach ulcers
- Support digestion and general bowel function
- Relieve pain and inflammation due to hemorrhoids
- Offer general anti-inflammatory benefits
- Contribute to some aspects of tissue healing and regeneration
- Confer nutritional protection against the development of some types of cancer
- Reduce the risk of periodontal disease and tooth decay
- Serve as a protective antioxidant, helping to protect the body from free-radical damage that may be associated with premature aging and degenerative disease
- Improve the body's utilization of essential fatty acids and protect them from oxidative damage
- Help address some of the symptoms associated with chronic fatigue syndrome (CFS and CFIDS)
- Help relieve some of the symptoms associated with benign prostatic hypertrophy (prostate enlargement, also called BPH)
- Be beneficial in reducing the severity of some epileptic seizures
- Help protect against kidney disease and bladder infections and may contribute to dissolving kidney stones
- Help prevent some types of liver disease
- Support optimal function of the thyroid in regulating metabolism
- Promote weight loss by increasing the metabolic rate

Confusion and Controversy — Not All Saturated Fats Are Equal

Although many nutritionists, doctors, and other health professionals have described the myriad health benefits of coconut oil, and Bruce Fife, a naturopathic physician, and Joseph Mercola, an osteopathic physician, have pronounced coconut oil as the healthiest oil to choose, coconut oil consumption has been the subject of fiery debate. Here are the issues at the core of the controversy.

First, many rigorous scientific studies have determined that consumption of trans-fatty acids poses a risk to health. There is an irrefutable link between eating trans-fatty acids and elevated blood cholesterol and increased risk of heart disease. Called trans fats for short, these "bad" fats don't often occur naturally—they are produced when liquid fat (oil) is turned into solid fat through a chemical process called partial or complete hydrogenation. Adding to the confusion is the fact that trans fats are, by definition, unsaturated fats; they belong to the same group of healthy oils that includes omega-3, -6, and -9.

So, to help consumers distinguish good fats from bad ones, nutritionists and health professionals have advised us to entirely eliminate the harmful trans fats from our diets and sharply limit or avoid saturated fats in favor of a diet including the healthy unsaturated fats. In recent years, we've grown accustomed to hearing trans fats and saturated fats (or "sat" fats, for short) spoken in the same breath and maligned as equally unhealthy. In general, sat fats are animal fats—butter, cream, bacon, cheese, lard, shortening, and gravy are all high in sat fats, while unsaturated fats have vegetable origins—olive, corn, soy, safflower, and canola oils. But it turns out that equating the health effects of trans fats and sat fats is mistaken and misleading because all sat fats are not equally unhealthy.

Coconut oil is a sat fat but it is not a trans fat, and while it's true that some sat fats can raise blood cholesterol, many studies have confirmed that coconut oil does not increase blood cholesterol and may even help to reduce total cholesterol and favorably improve the ratio of good to bad cholesterol. So why did it receive the same bad press as trans fats?

Some food industry observers contend that efforts to smear coconut oil with the same broad brush used to condemn trans and sat fats was at least in part financially motivated. Even though coconut and palm oil accounted for a scant 4 percent of edible oils used in the United States compared with soybean oil at 70 percent, during the 1980s, the American Soybean Association sought to restrict or limit importation of coconut and palm oil to maintain, or perhaps even increase, its market domination. The domestic versus foreign oil wars heated up, with coconut and palm oils derisively termed foreign "tropical oils" that threatened to imperil the health and lives of unsuspecting Americans.

Nebraska industrialist and self-styled consumer advocate Phil Sokolof fanned the flames of this controversy. Over nearly two decades, the eighty-one-year-old multimillionaire spent about fifteen million dollars of his own money on full-page newspaper advertisements informing Americans about the dangers of trans fats and sat fats. Inspired by a heart attack at age forty-three that he attributed to an unhealthy diet, Sokolof's organization, Heart Savers, promulgated many important public health messages about the importance of healthy diets and regular exercise, but it also served to further demonize all sat fats.

Unfortunately, the American Soybean Association's efforts and Sokolof's campaign also inspired major food processors to reformulate their products so they no longer used foreign tropical oils and prompted them to shift to hydrogenated oils, which contain trans fat and were, arguably, poorer choices in terms of public health.

Sadly, the successful campaign waged to discredit the healthfulness of coconut oil was largely successful and the scientific evidence supporting it as a healthy dietary fat has only resurfaced in recent years. By 1988, experts at the Harvard University Medical School asserted that, "For the U.S. consumer, the use of coconut oil does not increase the role of heart disease." Other research has confirmed that coconut oil consumption reduces the risk of atherosclerosis—clogging, narrowing, and hardening of blood vessels—along with other degenerative conditions. Coconut oil helps to prevent bacterial, viral, and fungal infections and, unlike some saturated fats, it does not raise cholesterol.

Research Confirms that Coconut Oil Is a Heart-Healthy Fat

Since coconut oil is a fat, you may be surprised to learn that a diet high in coconut oil has not been found to raise total blood cholesterol or low-density lipoprotein (LDL is often referred to as the bad cholesterol since elevated levels of this lipid are associated with increased risk for heart disease). When researchers compared diets rich in butter, coconut oil, and safflower oil, they found that cholesterol synthesis, total blood cholesterol, and LDL levels were lower among persons eating diets rich in coconut and safflower oils compared with those consuming diets rich in butter.

Researchers in Norway looked at the effect of diets rich in coconut oil on blood lipids, especially Lp(a), a lipoprotein that appears to be a risk factor for developing heart disease, and circulating tissue plasminogen activator antigen (t-PA antigen)—a long name for a blood marker that when elevated may indicate impaired glucose tolerance or type 2 diabetes. They found that diets rich in coconut oil reduced both t-PA antigen, Lp(a), and did not elevate blood lipids compared to diets rich in unsaturated fats.

Another study, performed using laboratory animals, found that coconut oil reduced total cholesterol, triglycerides, phospholipids, LDL and VLDL (very-low-density lipoproteins), and increased HDL (known as the good cholesterol, high-density lipoprotein is a protein in blood plasma that promotes breakdown and removal of cholesterol from the body). The researchers attributed coconut oil's beneficial effects on blood lipids to its biologically active polyphenol compounds. Polyphenols are naturally occurring chemical compounds that exert powerful antioxidant actions.

Cross-cultural and population studies produced more compelling evidence. Epidemiologists—scientists who consider the distribution of health and disease in populations rather than individuals—observed that cultures that consumed coconut oil such as the Polynesians, Sri Lankans, and Filipinos in general, had lower levels of blood cholesterol and heart disease when compared to other cultures.

Can Coconut Oil Help You Lose Weight?

If you're like most people who have struggled to diet and lose weight, your answer to this question is most likely to be, "fat chance!" Although it seems intuitively unlikely that eating fat could help you to lose fat, it turns out that there's some pretty persuasive evidence that people who get enough fat in their diets eat less and feel more satisfied than dieters who sharply reduce their fat intake.

While all fats naturally suppress appetite by prolonging satiety—primarily by slowing the emptying of the stomach—some are better than others at promoting weight loss. Some weight-loss experts recommend medium-chain triglycerides (MCTs contain fatty-acid chains that are 6 to 12 carbon atoms long) such as coconut and palm oils as opposed to long-chain triglycerides (LCTs contain more than 12 carbons per fatty acid) such as corn, soybean, safflower, and canola oils.

Unlike other fats, coconut oil is rapidly used by the body to produce energy rather than being stored as fat, in part because the body processes MCTs differently from other fats. Enzymes in the saliva and gastric juices break down MCTs almost entirely so there is little need for pancreatic enzymes to further digest them. As a result, people who suffer from digestive and metabolic problems can readily absorb MCTs compared with other fats that may traverse their systems incompletely or be only partially digested. Digestion of MCTs involves a breakdown to their individual component fatty acids, enabling them to be metabolized in much the same way as carbohydrates to produce a ready source of energy.

A large body of research demonstrates that when dieters replace LCTs with MCTs, they experience reduced appetite, increased thermogenesis—the body's ability to burn excess food to prevent weight gain—increased metabolism as measured by energy expenditure, reduced fat mass, and improved preservation of lean muscle mass.

One rigorous study—a double-blind, controlled-research protocol—compared the health benefits of MCTs versus LCTs on seventy-eight healthy volunteers over the course of twelve weeks. The study participants' weight and body fat were measured during weeks four, eight, and twelve. The fat, protein, and carbohydrate intakes did not differ significantly between the groups, yet among subjects who were overweight, as measured by body mass index (BMI), weight loss and body fat loss were significantly greater among those consuming the MCTs.

Coconut Oil for Healthy, Luminous Skin

There is no question that the Polynesian culture and others that include coconut oil in their diets have beautiful, clear, luminous skin. For years, coconut oil has been a staple ingredient in soaps and cosmetics aimed at nourishing skin so that it remains healthy, supple, and smooth.

When coconut oil is applied to the skin, it can form a chemical barrier that inhibits some types of infection. It has been used to relieve dryness and flaking and to prevent wrinkling, sagging skin, and age spots. It also protects the skin from some ultraviolet radiation damage.

While coconut oil may be responsible for the glowing skin of people living in tropical regions, it also has a role in treating skin conditions including cuts, burns, and psoriasis—a chronic skin disease characterized by periodic flare-ups that produce red patches covered with white scales. Like many other chronic diseases, psoriasis is believed to result from a combination of genetic and environmental factors—abnormalities in immune system function triggered by an environmental factor such as emotional stress, exposure to cold temperatures, injury, illness or infection, steroids and other medications, as well as mechanical stress such as constant pressure on the skin as a result of sitting or kneeling or skin exposure to chemicals.

There are many anecdotal and several published reports of using coconut oil to relieve symptoms of psoriasis, rashes, eczema, and rosacea. One published article asserts that coconut oil not only effectively treats symptoms of psoriasis but also seborrheic dermatitis and atopic dermatitis involving the scalp. It also cites coconut oil's ability to penetrate the hair shaft, protecting it from damage.

Since coconut oil has antifungal properties, it's not surprising that there are reports that it relieves symptoms of athlete's foot and jock itch, since fungi cause both. A natural lubricant, it makes an excellent massage oil, skin moisturizer, hair conditioner, and lip balm. Because coconut oil is effective against yeast, some women use it as a vaginal cream to soothe inflamed skin.

Although many people swear by using coconut oil topically, research suggests that to get the most benefits, it should be ingested as well as rubbed on the skin. Adding coconut oil to your diet is thought to form a continuously renewing layer of protection for your skin, defending it from potentially harmful pathogens.

What's in It?

Coconut oil is either liquid or a white solid, depending on the temperature. On a warm summer day—when the temperature reaches a balmy 76 degrees Fahrenheit—it pours easily from a jar. Stored in a cool cabinet, it becomes a white solid that practically melts at the touch, turning to liquid as soon as you rub it onto warm skin or heat it to stir-fry fresh vegetables.

About half of the fatty acids in coconut oil are lauric acid, a medium-chain fatty acid with 12 carbons and no double bonds. Coconut oil also contains capric acid, a medium-chain saturated fatty acid with 10 carbons and no double bonds. In the body, lauric acid forms monolaurin and capric acid forms monocaprin. This happens when saliva or bacteria on the skin break down the lauric acid or capric acid triglyceride into single units—since "mono" means one, the products of this breakdown are known as monolaurin and monocaprin. Both compounds are recognized for their ability to inhibit the growth of disease-causing microbes.

Lauric acid is known for its antimicrobial properties and the monoglyceride derivative of lauric acid, called monolaurin, is a potent antimicrobial that has demonstrated activity against a broad range of pathogens (disease-causing agents). Monolaurin has been found to be antibacterial, antiviral, and effective against many pathogenic protozoa. Interestingly, lauric acid occurs naturally in coconut milk and breast milk. The lauric acid in coconut oil is converted in the body to make the same disease-fighting fatty-acid-derivative monolaurin that infants make from the lauric acid they receive from breast milk. The monolaurin that infants make from breast milk or coconut-based formula serves to confer immunity and prevents them from contracting viral, bacterial, or protozoal infections.

Similarly, the monoglyceride derivative of capric acid is known as monocaprin, and it too has demonstrated antimicrobial action, particularly against *Chlamydia trachomatis* and

Neisseria gonorrhoeae, the culprits involved in many cases of sexually transmitted disease. Capric acid has also demonstrated the ability to swiftly and effectively eradicate three strains of *Candida albicans.*

The Center for Research on Lauric Oils, Inc., reports that some of the microorganisms that may be inactivated by lauric acid and monolaurin include lipid-coated viruses and bacteria. Examples of lipid-coated viruses include HIV, measles virus, herpes viruses, cytomegalovirus, Epstein–Barr, influenza, leukemia virus, pneumonovirus, rubeola virus, and sarcoma virus. Examples of lipid-coated bacteria are *Listeria monocytogenes, Heliobacter pylori* (gram negative), *Staphylococcus aureus, Streptococcus agalactiae,* and groups A, B, F, and G *streptococci.* Monolaurin also has been shown to inactivate several species of ringworm, *Candida albicans,* and *Giardia lamblia.*

Scientists believe that the antiviral action of monolaurin is largely attributable to its ability to disrupt and "dissolve" the lipoprotein envelope, or plasma membrane, that contains the virus. When it disrupts the lipid membrane it inactivates the virus by preventing attachment to the host's cell walls, effectively eliminating its ability to infect the host's cells.

Monolaurin's antimicrobial properties also may be the result of its ability to interfere with the pathogens' chemical communication systems and their ability to grow and multiply. It inhibits the replication of viruses by interrupting the binding of virus to host cells and prevents the uncoating of viruses necessary for them to replicate and cause infection. By binding to the envelope of the virus, monolaurin renders the virus more susceptible to the host's defenses.

Jigsaw Puzzle Science—
The Chemistry of Lipids

Lipids, like those found in coconut oil, comprise a family of organic chemicals that includes all oils, fats, and waxes. Chemically, all lipids are closely related by their chemical structure. The simplest way to understand how they are different is that oils are liquid at room temperature, fats are solid but have a low melting point, while waxes, like beeswax, the paraffin in candles, and lanolin from sheep's wool, are solid at room temperature but have a higher melting point than fats, usually quoted as more than 113 degrees Fahrenheit (45 degrees Celsius).

What all lipids have in common is that they are made up of long chains of carbon atoms surrounded, in various configurations, by hydrogen atoms. Lipids therefore belong to a large class of substances built around "hydrocarbons."

Putting Together the Pieces

While this talk about carbon and hydrogen and chains may seem pretty abstract, it's exactly like putting together a simple jigsaw puzzle made out of countless identical pieces that all fit together in certain very predictable ways.

Carbon atoms are the universal structural backbone of all organic chemicals. That's true because they are like a jigsaw puzzle piece with four "hooks" that look something like this:

The two hooks on the sides—one pointing out and one dimpling in, can link up, side to side, with other carbon atoms to form a chain, like this:

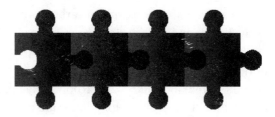

The essential properties of all lipids—including their physical characteristics like melting point and viscosity along with how they affect our health—are determined by:

- The length of their carbon chains
- The position of the hydrogen atoms around the chain
- Possible gaps where hydrogen atoms are missing, allowing the chain to bend
- Optional chemical groups, such as phosphates, that may be attached to the chain
- The way these chains are clustered together into larger groups, such as attaching to a glycerol molecule to become mono-, di-, and triglycerides

The Long and the Short of It— And a Lifesaving Oil

These hydrocarbon chains can be quite long. When they serve as the backbones of biological lipids in the body, they are usually not longer than sixteen or so carbons in length. Acetic acid, the chemical we know of as vinegar, is actually a very short chain fatty acid that's only two carbons in length. It's so short and chemically flexible that it doesn't seem to be oily at all!

Outside of the body, in other types of organic chemicals such as tar—a gooey black petroleum sludge churned out by oil refineries as they separate out the light, volatile, and economically valuable chemicals like gasoline and diesel fuel—the organic chains can be many thousands of carbons long.

Towards the longer end of the spectrum of biological lipids, a 16-carbon lipid chain called palmitic acid is the primary fat found in butter. There are even some very long chain fatty acids (called VLCFAs) in the body, like a 26-carbon molecule called hexacosanoic acid, but these super-long lipids are usually only minor players in the body's natural lipid environment.

Even though VLCFAs exist only in relatively small quantities in the body, it's nonetheless essential that we have the ability to process them. Some rare individuals have a genetic disorder, called adrenoleukodystrophy (or ALD for short), in which the ability to break down these very long chain lipids is absent. If you've seen the film *Lorenzo's Oil* you know the devastating consequences of this deficiency.

The film is based on the deeply moving true-life story of Augusto Odone, whose young son Lorenzo is crippled by ALD—a condition that devastates the production of myelin, the fatty coating around our nerves. Told by every doctor he visits that there is no way to relieve his beloved Lorenzo of his horrific pain and suffering, Augusto decides to study organic chemistry—a field totally new and alien to him. Driven by his love for his son and his complete freedom from medical dogma, he actually discovers a way to make a new kind of oil—dubbed Lorenzo's Oil—that can at least partially compensate for his son's inability to break down VLCFAs.

Lorenzo's Oil is good drama, good science, and even good business. Augusto Odone was granted a United States patent for the manufacture of Lorenzo's Oil and all profits are donated to a charitable organization, the Myelin Foundation, which conducts research seeking a cure for profound disturbances of lipid metabolism.

The Fatty-Acid Test

You may have noticed that the word *acid* appears in each of these chemicals' names—after all, we've been referring to them as "fatty-acid chains." While we usually think of acids as corrosive liquids like hydrochloric acid that foams and fumes and burns through steel doors in action movies, to a chemist all it means for something to be an acid is that it has an extra hydrogen atom that it gives away when it enters into a chemical reaction. When an acid donates a hydrogen atom, it opens up a hook that can be used to attach the acid to another chemical group. In a little while, when we look at our jigsaw puzzle's representation of a lipid, you'll see that there is just such an extra hydrogen waiting to drop off and create a molecular connecting hook.

Now, you'll notice that the carbon chain also has jigsaw puzzle hooks on the top and bottom as well. In the biological carbon chains within our bodies, most of these hooks are linked to hydrogen atoms. But if you hooked a long carbon chain up with fluorine atoms instead of hydrogen you'd get a chemical technically referred to as polytetrafluoroethylene. It's an intimidating mouthful of a name, but you and I know it better as Teflon—the non-stick coating used on pots and pans. (Teflon is a registered trademark of E. I. du Pont de Nemours and Company.)

Let's take a look at our simple 4-carbon-chain jigsaw puzzle with hydrogen atoms attached. Each of the little "hats" above and below the carbon chain represents an atom of hydrogen. I've put "C" and "H" on the carbons and hydrogens to help you keep track:

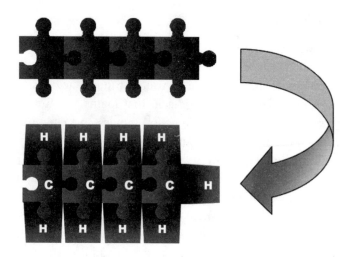

Notice how all of the up and down hooks on the original carbon chain (above) are all linked to hydrogens (below). There's even a hydrogen all the way on the right side acting like a cap that closes off the chain.

This capped area at the right is called the *omega* end of the carbon chain, since omega is the last letter of the Greek alphabet, and this capped carbon is the last one in the chain. (It's a given in life that scientists like to use obscure symbols to name simple things.) But this one is important. You may have heard that omega-3, omega-6, and omega-9 oils are important to your health. In a moment, we're going to see exactly what that means. By the way, it shouldn't come as a surprise that the other end of the chain, at the left side of our picture, is called the alpha end of the chain.

In our picture, the carbon hook at the alpha end is still unfilled. For your basic fatty-acid chain, that final position is capped with a molecular group called carboxyl—two oxygens with one hydrogen hanging off the end. One technical detail that you can ignore (but I've added it into the picture) is that one of the oxygens has a double bond with the carbon—that

just means that they bond using two of the carbon atom's hooks. Don't worry about it.... I'm just striving for accuracy in the event that any chemists may read this!

Here's what the whole fatty-acid jigsaw puzzle looks like, in all its glory:

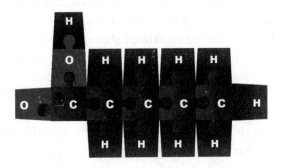

The strip of jigsaw puzzle pieces in the center are our original carbons, forming the backbone of the chain, with hydrogen atoms linked above, below, and at the omega end on the right. The new block, on the left at the alpha end, contains the final carbon linked with two oxygen atoms—shown in gray—and one more hydrogen on top. That last carbon atom has both an "innie" and an "outie" link because it's double bonded to the oxygen on the left ... but that's the detail you can ignore.

That's it—a free fatty-acid chain jigsaw puzzle. Not too difficult, right?

The Fatty Acids Get Hitched

There are a few more pieces of the puzzle we should consider if you're really interested in understanding the chemistry of lipids. You've probably heard of triglycerides. Often, when you get a medical checkup, your doctor will order a blood lipids profile that gives you information about how much cholesterol and other lipids are present in your blood.

Too much buildup of fat in the blood can contribute to heart disease and various other inflammatory conditions. Modern medicine also distinguishes between "good" and "bad" blood lipids called HDLs, or high-density lipoproteins, and LDLs and VLDLs, or low- and very-low-density lipoproteins. A lipoprotein is a special kind of molecule that forms when a lipid connects with a protein. The ratio of good HDLs to bad LDLs and VLDLs is an important marker of cardiovascular health.

Triglycerides are molecules that contain three fatty-acid chains like the one we illustrated above. Diglycerides contain two chains, and monoglycerides have only one chain. The "glyceride" part of the description refers to a 3-carbon molecule, called glycerol, that acts as a "hitching post" where one, two, or three fatty-acid chains can attach. When we consume fats and oils in foods, they're usually in this glyceride form.

Part of our metabolic biochemistry transforms glycerides into free fatty-acid chains by unhooking them from the glycerol hitching post. Other parts of our fatty-acid metabolism then take these chains apart, rearrange them, and convert them into the many forms our bodies need. One of these forms, called coenzyme A (or just CoA for short), is the primary fuel used by most of our cells to produce energy. Other forms get connected to other molecules and are used to make essential substances like hormones, which are chemical messengers that flow through the body and control critical physiological processes, or myelin, the sheaths that insulate and protect our nerves, or phospholipids that serve as the primary components of the vital membranes surrounding each of our cells. (See Cells, Lipids, and the Biology of Self below.)

Without going into too much more detail, we can simply note that there is a process for hitching fatty-acid chains onto the glycerol molecule and a reverse process for unhitching them. By the way, when we unhitch all the fatty-acid chains from a glycerol molecule, the leftover glycerol gets converted into glucose—the primary cellular fuel used by our hearts and our brains. Waste not, want not!

An interesting note is that the fatty acids in a triglyceride molecule can all be the same or they can be different. Also, most naturally occurring fats contain a complex combination of triglycerides that mix and match different fatty acids. Part of our perception of the greasiness of fatty foods arises from the fact that these different fats all melt at different temperatures. One exception is cocoa butter, the lipid used as the base for making chocolate. Cocoa butter mostly contains the same triglyceride configuration, meaning that all its components melt at the same temperature. This is a major factor in our perception of chocolate as silky and smooth when it melts in our mouths, rather than greasy.

Cells, Lipids, and the Biology of Self

You've probably heard the old expression that oil and water don't mix. While it's certainly true that chemically oil and water repel one another, the expression is usually meant in a more philosophical way, to describe people of different temperaments who just can't get along. But the antagonistic relationship between oil and water is profound in another way. The chemical reality that oil and water don't mix is actually the structural basis for all cellular life on Earth.

If you've ever looked through a microscope at living tissue, even just a few cells gently scraped away from your own cheek with a toothpick, you could see that each cell has a membrane, a kind of biological fence that holds all the parts in. It makes sense—if there wasn't some sort of fence, all the parts would slide out and there wouldn't be any distinction between "inside" and "outside." It's hard to imagine what kind of living things could exist if they didn't have some kind of a boundary. In essence, our cellular membranes separate what is "us"—the stuff on the inside—from what is "other"—all the stuff on the outside.

Now, if we take a good look at the cell's membrane, we notice something really fascinating. Chemically, it's mostly made of lipids—the oils and fats we've just been talking about.

And oil doesn't mix with water, right? But there's a little twist. Each of the lipid molecules has an extra chemical group at the end, called a phosphate, which actually attracts water! That's intriguing, because we now have a molecule that attracts water on one end—the phosphate end—and repels water at the other end—the lipid end. The phospholipid, as such a molecule is called, is sort of like a magnet except that instead of having a north pole and a south pole, it has a "hydrophilic" (water-loving) pole and a "hydrophobic" (water-avoiding) pole.

Here's where it gets interesting. Every cell is really a tiny drop of seawater wrapped up in a skin. The skin, called the cellular membrane, is made out of countless pairs of phospholipid molecules. One phospholipid from each pair has a water-attracting head that faces inward, towards the drop of water inside the cell, while the hydrophilic phosphate head of the other phospholipid faces outward—towards the watery environment that bathes the cell from the outside, whether that water is in blood, lymph, or another biological fluid. Both of the hydrophobic lipid tails face each other, avoiding the water.

Put it all together and here's what a cellular membrane— sometimes called a phosholipid bilayer membrane—looks like. The bilayer membrane is an amazing feat of molecular engineering where the simple fact that oil and water don't mix gives rise to the most fundamental distinction that our cells can make: what belongs to us, on the inside, and what belongs to the rest of the world, on the outside.

Now, if every cell in the body derives it integrity—its very knowledge of "self"—from the fats and oils in its membrane, it's not a big stretch to see that the health of every cell is dependent, in part, on the quality of the dietary lipids that we consume. As we've already seen, coconut oil is a healthy lipid possessing many properties that make it ideal for cooking and for use as a nutritional supplement.

Dr. Bruce Lipton, a leading cellular biologist, goes a step further. He believes that most of the incredible biological intelligence of the cell resides not in its DNA—the so-called "molecule of life" that has dominated biology since the discovery of its structure in 1953—but in the cell membrane. He points to the fact that the membrane is exactly the right thickness to hold special embedded molecules called integral membrane proteins (IMPs) that act as sensory organs and robotic arms, helping the cell to be aware of its environment and to respond intelligently and adeptly.

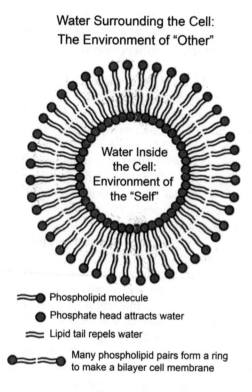

Water Surrounding the Cell:
The Environment of "Other"

Water Inside
the Cell:
Environment of
the "Self"

—● Phospholipid molecule
● Phosphate head attracts water
≈ Lipid tail repels water
●——● Many phospholipid pairs form a ring
to make a bilayer cell membrane

Traditional biological theory describes transactions between the cell's interior environment—the cellular *cytoplasm*—and the exterior environment around the cell in terms of "channels" and other constructs. In fact, these so-called channels don't really exist—they are actually a sort of after-the-fact description of the incredibly adept molecular activities choreographed by the cell membrane and its host of embedded IMPs.

Remember, these intelligent proteins only work because they are properly situated in the lipids that make up our cellular membranes.

In his recent book *The Biology of Belief*, Lipton extends this idea much further. Because the biological behavior of cells—and therefore our very life and health—is conditioned by the environment and because our perception of the environment is strongly influenced by our minds, ultimately our beliefs and perceptions have direct control over our health.

The following is a quote from Dr. Lipton's Web site that puts this leading-edge science into perspective:

> The functional units of life are the individual cells that comprise our bodies. Though every cell is innately intelligent and can survive on its own when removed from the body, in the body, each cell foregoes its individuality and becomes a member of a multicellular community. The body really represents the cooperative effort of a community of perhaps fifty trillion single cells. By definition, a community is an organization of individuals committed to supporting a shared vision. Consequently, while every cell is a free-living entity, the body's community accommodates the wishes and intents of its "central voice," a character we perceive as the mind and spirit.
>
> When the mind perceives that the environment is safe and supportive, the cells are preoccupied with the growth and maintenance of the body. In stressful situations, cells forego their normal growth functions and adopt a defensive "protection" posture. The body's energy resources normally used to sustain growth are diverted to systems that provide protection during periods of stress. Simply, growth processes are restricted or suspended in a stressed system. While our systems can accommodate periods of acute (brief) stress, prolonged or chronic stress is debilitating for its energy demands interfere with the required maintenance of the body, and as a consequence, leads to dysfunction and disease.

"Sat Fat"—You Want Fries with That?

Another important distinction we've noted and you've probably heard about is the difference between saturated and unsaturated fats. You may have even heard more detailed descriptions of monounsaturated and polyunsaturated fats. Now that you know the jigsaw puzzle chemistry of fatty-acid chains it's easy to explain what these terms mean.

As we mentioned earlier, saturated fats have gotten a bad rap, being associated with various types of coronary heart disease. But recently, researchers are recognizing that some saturated fats, like those found in coconut oil, are actually healthful and that many of the dangers associated with saturated fat are really the result of a distortion in the position of hydrogen atoms around the carbon chain as they form something known as "trans fat," which we'll describe in just a moment.

Some trans fats form naturally, but most of this unhealthful substance is created when oils are heated to high temperatures. This can happen during cooking—like making french fries in a fast-food restaurant—or when manufacturers heat and chemically transform liquid oils to make them into solid products like margarine through a process called hydrogenation. One of the great benefits of coconut oil is that it can be used for cooking at moderately high temperatures without forming unhealthy trans fat molecules.

Remember, to build the lipid molecule we started with a string of carbon atoms joined side to side to form a chain. Each carbon then got linked, top and bottom, with a hydrogen atom. The hook at the far end, the so-called omega end of the chain, also got capped off with a hydrogen, while the alpha end got attached to a carbon-oxygen-hydrogen group that could hitch and unhitch it from a glycerol molecule. That's all you need to remember to understand saturation.

A saturated lipid is simply one in which every available carbon hook is linked to a hydrogen atom. In other words, in saturated lipids there are no gaps in the chain. If you think about it, it makes sense that saturated fats tend to be solid—like butter and lard—since the carbon chain is completely filled in. Without any gaps in the chain there are no places where the molecule can bend. Something that can't bend is going to be stiff and solid.

Conversely, an *un*saturated lipid is one that has one or more gaps where some of the hydrogens that could have been linked are absent. When this happens, the adjacent carbon atoms form a double bond with one another, using two hooks to hold each other rather than the usual one hook.

Now, if a fatty-acid chain has a gap in it—or maybe even two or three gaps where hydrogen atoms are missing—that means there are places where the carbon chain can bend. If the chain can bend then it's flexible rather than stiff. On a macroscopic level, the flexible lipid will act as a liquid instead of a solid.

Fatty acids with one missing pair of adjacent hydrogen atoms, like the one shown in this illustration, are called *monounsaturated* lipids because there's one place where the carbon chain isn't filled up—or saturated—with hydrogens and can therefore bend. If the fatty-acid chain has two or more gaps it's referred to as a *polyunsaturated* lipid.

Omega Oils

Now, what about the omega-3 and -6 and -9 oils that we hear so much about? Simple. An unsaturated lipid is named for the *first gap* where hydrogen atoms are missing from the chain, counting *backward* from the omega end. If the first missing hydrogen gap is, say, 3 carbons back from the omega end of the chain then it's called an omega-3 fatty acid. If the first gap is 6 carbons back from the end of the chain, it's an omega-6, and so forth.

Physiologically, the placement of the gap—whether a lipid has an omega-3, -6, or -9 configuration—turns out to be very important. Surprisingly, research shows that in some ways the *ratios* between our intake of these essential fatty acids may have more of an impact on our health than the amounts of the oils themselves. This is because their relative proportions in our system shift which chemical reactions are most likely to take place. This not only has impact on our metabolism and utilization of fatty acids as cellular fuel, but also affects the formation of hormones and other important biochemicals that govern many processes including inflammatory and anti-inflammatory responses.

Whose Side Are You On, Anyway?
Cis-Fats Versus Trans Fats

The natural configuration of hydrogen atoms around a gap in an unsaturated lipid is for both of the hydrogens to be on the same side of the chain. This is referred to as the cis- configuration because *cis* is a Latin word meaning "on the same side." Here's a simple picture of a carbon double bond somewhere along a cis-fatty-acid chain where two hydrogen atoms are missing. Both of the hydrogens that are present are on the same side of the chain.

$$\begin{matrix} \text{H} & & \text{H} \\ | & & | \\ \text{-C} & = & \text{C-} \end{matrix}$$

When unsaturated fat and oils are heated to a sufficient degree, the bonds holding the hydrogen atoms in place are weakened and parts of the molecule can slip around, changing places. Often, one of the hydrogen atoms winds up on the other side of the carbon chain. This is referred to as the trans- configuration. *Trans* in Latin means, "on the opposite side." Fats that swap their hydrogen atoms around like this are called trans-fatty acids (or just "trans fats" for short), and they pose a significant risk to our health.

Here's a simple picture of a trans-fatty configuration. You can clearly see that the two hydrogens straddle the carbon chain—with one on each side.

$$\begin{matrix} \text{H} & & \\ | & & \\ \text{-C} & = & \text{C-} \\ & & | \\ & & \text{H} \end{matrix}$$

Consumption of trans fats increases the levels of LDL and VLDL, the "bad cholesterol" in the body. It has also been shown to lower the level of HDL, the "good cholesterol" therefore worsening the critical HDL/LDL ratio. Trans fat is believed to contribute to the development of atherosclerotic plaque and also may play a role in the development of obesity, metabolic syndrome, and diabetes.

Trans fats also are associated with elevated levels of C-reactive protein (CRP), an inflammatory immune system chemical that is often used as a predictive marker for cardiovascular distress. The high-temperature cooking processes that produce some of the trans fats we eat are also associated with the creation of advanced glycation endproducts (AGEs). These are basically "crusts" of sugar molecules that attach to proteins and form stiff cross-linkages. These linkages degrade our tissues and accelerate the aging process—both on the inside, by diminishing the functional capacity of our organs, and on the outside, by promoting visible wrinkles and dry and sagging skin.

Finally, some researchers are concerned that when trans-fatty acids become integrated into cell membranes they may alter important structures essential to cellular health. We looked at the fact that the cell membrane is thought to be the seat of the cell's native intelligence and that it has just the right structure to support an array of integral membrane proteins that provide a host of incredibly sophisticated services.

The integration of trans fat into these membranes may interfere with these functions, essentially "dumbing down" the cell to the point where it can no longer function in an optimal fashion. Some researchers are also concerned that expectant mothers who have diets high in trans fats may be loading the cells of their unborn children with poorly functioning building blocks, potentially setting the stage for future health problems.

A Complete Breakdown of the Nutrients in Coconut Oil

Nutrient	Units	Value per 100 grams
Proximates		
Energy	kcal	862
Energy	kj	3607
Total lipid (fat)	g	100.00
Minerals		
Iron, Fe	mg	0.04
Vitamins		
Vitamin E (alpha-tocopherol)	mg	0.09
Tocopherol, gamma	mg	0.20
Vitamin K (phylloquinone)	mcg	0.5
Lipids		
Fatty acids, total saturated	g	86.500
6:0	g	0.600
8:0	g	7.500
10:0	g	6.000
12:0	g	44.600
14:0	g	16.800
16:0	g	8.200
18:0	g	2.800
Fatty acids, total monounsaturated	g	5.800
18:1 undifferentiated	g	5.800
Fatty acids, total polyunsaturated	g	1.800
18:2 undifferentiated	g	1.800
Phytosterols	mg	86

USDA National Nutrient Database for Standard Reference, Release 18 (2005)

The Many Uses of Coconut Oil

Coconut oil can be used in an almost endless variety of ways. It can be taken directly, straight out of the bottle, as a nutritional supplement. Many people have reported remarkable improvement of their arthritis and other inflammatory conditions when they take several tablespoons of coconut oil daily.

Coconut oil may be applied to the body to keep skin soft and supple. Used this way, it also protects the skin from infections and blocks some harmful ultraviolet radiation. Liquid coconut oil may also be used as a lubricant for massage, either in its natural form, or with a small amount of essential oil, such as lavender or ylang-ylang added for a gentle, soothing fragrance.

Some scientists have even proposed making a diesel fuel, called Coco Biodiesel, out of coconut oil. Coco Biodiesel is less polluting than gasoline and conventional diesel fuel. Added to ordinary gasoline, even in very small amounts, it has been shown to reduce particulate emissions, thereby reducing air pollution.

It's Easy to Add Coconut Oil to Your Diet

The best part of this nutrition advice is that it's news you can use. It's easier to change your cooking oil than your car oil—and better for your health. Coconut oil can be used to safely fry foods at moderately high temperatures without the risk of creating damaging trans fats. Stir-fry, sauté, and broil with coconut oil—it's light and doesn't overpower fresh vegetables. Many people actually prefer fragrant coconut oil with its subtle nutty taste to other vegetable oils. The only place you won't want to substitute it is in cold salads, since the liquid oil will solidify when tossed with cold vegetables.

Coconut oil becomes solid when refrigerated or when the temperature falls below 76 degrees Fahrenheit, its freezing point. In its soft, semi-solid state, coconut oil makes an excellent spread, in place of butter on freshly baked, whole-grain bread or crackers. In baking, coconut oil is an excellent stand-in for butter, margarine, or shortening. Breads, cakes, and muffins made with coconut oil are light, moist, and healthy.

Coconut oil also makes an excellent dairy substitute in hot drinks, giving coffee, Postum, or herbal tea a rich, creamy flavor. Blend it into shakes and smoothies as well.

Many cookbooks contain inventive, tasty ways to use coconut oil. *The Good Fat Cookbook* by Fran McCullough (New York: Scriber, 2003) and *Nourishing Traditions: The Cookbook that Challenges Politically Correct Nutrition and the Diet Dictocrats,* 2nd ed., by Sally Fallon and Mary Enig (Winona Lake, IN: New Trends Publishing, 1999) both contain a wealth of terrific recipes using coconut oil.

References

Bergsson, G., et al. "In vitro killing of *Candida albicans* by fatty acids and monoglycerides. *Antimicrob Agents Chemother.* 2001; 45(11): 3209–12.

The Biology of Belief: Unleashing The Power Of Consciousness, Matter And Miracles. Santa Rosa, CA: Mountain of Love/Elite Publishing, 2005.

Cox, C., et al. "Effects of dietary coconut oil, butter, and safflower oil on plasma lipids, lipoproteins and lathosterol levels." *European Journal of Clinical Nutrition.* 1998; 52:650–54.

Dayrit, C. S. "Coconut Oil in Health and Disease: Monolaurin's Potential as Cure for HIV/AIDS." Department of Health, Republic of the Philippines (http://www.doh.gov.ph/SARS/coconut_ oil.htm)

Enig, M. G. "Coconut Oil: An Anti-bacteria, Anti-viral Ingredient for Food, Nutrition and Health." AVOC Lauric Symposium. Manila, Philippines, October 17, 1997.

Fife, B. *Eat Fat, Look Thin: A Safe and Natural Way to Lose Weight Permanently.* Colorado Springs, CO: Piccadilly Books, Ltd., 2002.

Hierholzer, J. C., Kabara, J. J. "In vitro effects of monolaurin compounds on enveloped RNA and DNA viruses." *Journal of Food Safety* 1982; 4(1): 1–12.

Hunter, B. T. "How a PR Campaign Led to Unhealthy Diets." *Consumer's Research* 2003; 86(8)http://www.coconutresearchcenter. org/article10027.htm.

Kabara, J. J. *Pharmacological Effects of Lipids*, Vols. 1–3. Champaign, IL: AOCS Press, 1990.

Komaroff, A. L. "By the Way, Doctor." *Harvard Medical Letter*, April 2006.

Lipton, B. H. "Uncovering the Biology of Belief" http://www.brucelipton.com/article/mind-over-genes-the-new-biology, accessed June 23, 2006.

Lim-Sylianco, C. Y. , et al. "A Comparison of Germ Cell Antigenotoxic Activity of Non-Dietary and Dietary Coconut Oil and Soybean Oil." *Phil. Journal of Coconut Studies.* 1992; XVII 2:6–10.

Muller, H., et al. "A Diet Rich in Coconut Oil Reduces Diurnal Postprandial Variations in Circulating Tissue Plasminogen Activator Antigen and Fasting Lipoprotein (a) compared with a Diet Rich in Unsaturated Fat in Women." *Journal of Nutrition.* 2003; 133(11): 3422–27.

Nevin, K. G., Rajamohan, T. "Beneficial effects of virgin coconut oil on lipid parameters and in vitro LDL oxidation." *Clinical Biochemistry* 2004; 37(9): 830–35.

St-Onge, M. P., Jones, P. J. H. "Physiological Effects of Medium-Chain Triglycerides: Potential Agents in the Prevention of Obesity." *Journal of Nutrition.* 2002; 132: 329–32.

St-Onge, M. P., et al. "Medium-Chain Triglycerides Increase Energy Expenditure and Decrease Adiposity in Overweight Men." *Obesity Research.* 2003; 11: 395–402.

Projan, S. J., et al. "Glycerol monolaurate inhibits the production of beta-lactamase, toxic shock toxin-1, and other staphylococcal exoproteins by interfering with signal transduction." *Journal of Bacteriology.* 1994; 176: 4204–09.

Shah, M. K. "Coconut oil compound ointment." *Indian J Dermatol Venereol Leprol* 2003; 69: 303–04.

Tayzag, E., et al. Monolaurin and Coconut Oil as Monotherapy for HIV-AIDS. Pilot Trial.

Tsuji, H., et al. "Dietary Medium-Chain Triacylglycerols Suppress Accumulation of Body Fat in a Double-Blind, Controlled Trial in Healthy Men and Women." *Journal of Nutrition.* 2001; 131: 2853–59.